Infection Control for the Dental Team

Quintessentials of Dental Practice – 39

Clinical Practice – 3

Infection Control for the Dental Team

By

Michael V Martin
Martin R Fulford
Antony J Preston

Editor-in-Chief: Nairn H F Wilson
Series Editor: Nairn H F Wilson

Quintessence Publishing Co. Ltd.
London, Berlin, Chicago, Paris, Milan, Barcelona, Istanbul,
São Paulo, Tokyo, New Delhi, Moscow, Prague, Warsaw

British Library Cataloguing in Publication Data
Martin, Michael (Michael V.)
Infection control for the dental team
1. Dentistry, Operative - Complications 2. Infection -
Prevention
I. Title II. Fulford, Martin R. III. Preston, Antony J.
617.6'05

ISBN-13: 9781850971320

ISBN-13: 978-1-85097-132-0

Foreword

Infection control is central to the clinical practice of dentistry. It is a responsibility of all members of the dental team, individually and collectively. Failures in standards of infection control may be the subject of legal actions, let alone actions in respect of professional conduct. Patients and the public at large must be protected from the unnecessary spread of infection and all members of the dental team must be safe in their working environment.

Infection Control for the Dental Team, a most important addition to the now near-complete *Quintessentials of Dental Practice* series, deals with infection control risk, medical histories and personal protection, surgery design and equipment, instrument decontamination, disinfection and ethical and legal responsibilities in infection control. In addition, this excellent volume concludes with most helpful models, policies, protocols and checklists for robust infection control arrangements. If you have any uncertainties about any aspect of infection control or wish to ensure compliance with legal requirements, let alone national and international guidance on infection control, this *Quintessentials* volume will address your needs.

In keeping with all the other volumes in the *Quintessentials* series, *Infection Control for the Dental Team* is succinct, engaging and capable of being read through in a few hours. It is anticipated, however, that this book will not just be read through, but will become a valuable training resource, important source of reference and highly regarded guidance on infection control for the dental practitioner and the dental team. And if that is not exceptional value for money, implementation of the guidance provided in this book will be good insurance in terms of being able to refute any allegations of failure in infection control.

All in all, another outstanding addition to the *Quintessentials* series. Congratulations to the authors on an important job well done, and to a very high standard.

Nairn Wilson
Editor-in-Chief

Preface

Infection control is part of every dental professional's daily practice. In this book we have attempted to offer the busy professional simple and effective guidance based on an accurate risk assessment. We have used this guidance to set working methods in a variety of different settings, from dental hospitals to practices, and found it to work without loss of clinical time. We have also included an extensive set of generic protocols that can be easily modified according to the needs of each particular clinical setting. Our hope is that this book will ensure that dental professionals have a safe and practical working environment that is free from the risk of transmitted infection.

MV Martin

MR Fulford

AJ Preston

Contents

Chapter 1
The Risks

Aim

The aim of this chapter is to describe the risks of contracting an infectious disease in the dental surgery environment.

Outcome

After reading this chapter, you should have a basic understanding of how infectious disease could potentially be transmitted in dentistry.

Terminology

Infection control in dentistry is all the methods we use to prevent the transmission of potentially pathogenic micro-organisms. The transmission of micro-organisms does not always result in infection. To cause an infection, the micro-organisms have to be transferred in sufficient numbers and then multiply to cause infectious disease. The number of bacteria, viruses, fungi or prions that are necessary to infect is called the *minimum infective dose*, as can be measured in experimental animals. The minimum infective dose can be decreased if a person's defence mechanisms are impaired, for example, by chronic long-standing debilitating disease, medical interventions (immunosuppressive drugs, cytotoxic therapy) or very rarely by congenital disease; such patients are described as being medically compromised or immunocompromised.

Potential Routes of Transmission of Infection

When dentistry was practised without the use of any protective barriers or effective decontamination, there was an increased potential for the transmission of infection by direct contact. The routine use of barrier methods has reduced this potential to almost nil. With the growth in world travel and the increase in hepatitis, HIV and tuberculosis, infection control in dentistry is all the more important.

Dental procedures often create aerosols containing water, blood and saliva.

The risk from the inhalation of aerosols by patients or dental personnel has never been completely or reliably assessed. The highest risk of transmission of infection is by direct blood-to-blood contact. This contact can occur through injuries by "sharps" that penetrate the epithelium or by direct inoculation of wounds by contaminated instruments. Another potential route of transmission is through the conjunctiva of the eye.

Potential Pathogens in Dentistry

Although potentially any micro-organism could cause infection in dentistry, in practice only a selected few have been proven to be involved. These are shown in Table 1-1. This is because the oral cavity and saliva are selective in the number and type of micro-organisms that are usually present. In addition, while blood could contain many pathogens, it is usually sterile. Nevertheless, it is wise to routinely presume that every patient is potentially infectious. The presumption that every patient is potentially infectious logically leads to use of a standard set of infection control methods; these are often called *universal* or standard precautions. The use of standard precautions for every patient has not been adopted by all dentists. In some countries different types of infection control precautions are used for different procedures; this is problematical as it presumes that patients can be accurately assessed as potential carriers of disease but this is often not possible.

Table 1-1 **Micro-organisms implicated in infection from dental treatment**

Micro-organism	Probable route of transmission
Herpes simplex type 1	Hands, record cards, splatter from oral cavity
Hepatitis B	Sharps injuries, trans-conjunctival
HIV	Possibly contaminated needles or local anaesthetic
Hand, foot and mouth disease	Direct contact with infected skin
Methicillin-resistant *Staphylococcus aureus*	Hands
Tuberculosis	Aerosols
Pseudomonas aeruginosa	Infected water lines, aerosols
Legionella pneumophila	Infected water lines, aerosols

Viruses

Potentially any virus could be transmitted by dental procedures, but those of greatest concern are the herpes and hepatitis viruses.

Hepatitis B was transmitted by dental procedures before the introduction of vaccines against this virus. Some of the transmissions of hepatitis B have resulted in the deaths of dental personnel. Most transmissions have been by blood-to-blood contact, usually following sharps injuries. Saliva could potentially transmit hepatitis as the concentration of the virus in saliva can be very high at certain stages of the illness. Transmission of hepatitis B has also been described through the conjunctiva of the eye.

Hepatitis C has been suspected to be transmitted in dentistry, but there is little evidence to support this contention. The virus has been found in the saliva of infected persons, but in concentrations well below the minimum infective dose. Recent research has also shown that even sharps injuries suffered by dental personnel with instruments used on carriers of hepatitis C have not resulted in transmission of this virus.

Human immunodeficiency virus (HIV) can be found in saliva but usually in low numbers. There have been extensive studies to determine if this virus could be transmitted by dental procedures. With one exception, no transmission has been proven. The exception is the curious case of Dr Acer, a practitioner in Florida, who was infected with HIV and who is thought to have transmitted the virus during dental procedures on five patients. This is an exceptional case.

Herpes simplex type 1 has been transmitted during dental procedures either by contact, or splashing of saliva into the eye. Infections have caused blindness in dental personnel who had not worn protective glasses during operative procedures. Herpetic hand whitlows (Fig 1-1) used to be common among dentists, but have almost been eradicated by the use of protective gloves. The minimum infective dose of herpes simplex type 1 is very low and thus *elective* dental treatment should not be done on patients who are developing or have herpetic perioral or intraoral lesions (cold sores).

Elective treatment of patients with oral herpes should be postponed until the lesions have completely healed. If emergency treatment is necessary on patients with oral herpetic lesions, then barrier precautions must be adopted and the minimum number of personnel should be involved in the procedures.

3

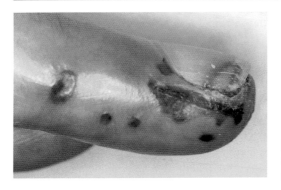

Fig 1-1 Herpetic whitlows caused by cross infection in a dental student.

Approximately 30% of the population get oral herpetic lesions caused by herpes simplex type 1, and almost 100% carry it commensally. Recent research has shown that the 30% who get oral herpetic infections shed the virus in high concentrations into saliva almost continually. The virus has a very low minimum infective dose and is the single most infectious agent dentists have to deal with in practice.

Hand, foot and mouth disease has been spread by direct contact principally in hospitals. This virus is very contagious but reports of its spread in dentistry have diminished to almost nil since the introduction of routine glove wearing.

Bacteria
A number of bacteria have been implicated as causes of cross infection in dentistry, including *Legionella* species and methicillin-resistant *Staphylococcus aureus* (MRSA).

Legionella pneumophilia has caused the death of one practitioner, probably as a result of inhalation of infected droplets from his dental unit water supply.

Similarly, *Pseudomonas aeruginosa* has caused two infections in medically compromised individuals, most likely again from infected water lines.

MRSA has been transmitted in dentistry probably by contact, by means of unprotected, contaminated hands.

By far the most important infection risk to dental personnel is tuberculosis.

The World Health Organization has estimated that one third of the world's population carry tuberculosis. The most common cause is strains of *Mycobacterium tuberculosis*. This bacterium is principally transmitted by aerosols, but it has been suggested that it could also be transmitted by contact with infected dental instruments.

Yeasts

The main yeast that has been implicated in transmission of infection by dental procedures is *Candida albicans*. There is evidence that this yeast has been spread from the mouths of neonates to others by direct contact.

Prions

Prions are proteins that cause transmissible spongiform encephalopathies, including Creutzfeldt-Jakob disease. Whether prions can be transmitted by dental procedures is still not fully determined, but the likelihood is that they are not. Prions have been found in various oral tissues, but there is no evidence that they get into the oral cavity or saliva. Prions stick tenaciously to stainless steel and their potential presence has led to improvements in pre-sterilisation cleaning (see Chapter 4).

The Future Risks

The expansion of world travel has meant that people are mobile and disease is readily spread to new places. For example, haemorrhagic fevers have been seen in Europe where previously they were almost exclusively confined to sub-Saharan Africa. Fortunately, these diseases have never been spread by dental procedures.

In addition, new diseases may develop by mutation. A good example is severe acute respiratory syndrome (SARS), which is spread by close contact and droplets. SARS is a mutated common-cold virus.

Another potential threat is avian flu virus. If this virus were to acquire genes from the human influenza virus, thereby allowing it to infect humans, then a global pandemic would result. Since avian flu would be spread by close contact and droplet infection, dentistry would be a potential risk.

These new diseases reinforce the need for constant surveillance of infectious diseases and for the dental profession to react to their threats in a measured way, based on the available science.

Conclusions

- A variety of bacteria, viruses and yeasts can potentially be transmitted by dental procedures.
- The safest means of preventing the transmission of infection in dentistry is to use standard precautions for infection control.

Further reading

Bagg J, Macfarlane TW, Poxton IR, Miller CH, Smith AJ. Essentials of Microbiology for Dental Students, ed 2. Oxford: Oxford University Press, 2004.

Lamey PJ, Lewis MA. Oral medicine in practice: viral infection. Br Dent J 1989;167:269–274.

Lassiter TE, Panagakos FS. Tuberculosis. NY State Dent J 2003;69:23–26.

Whitworth C. vCJD and dental treatment: where are we now? Prim Dent Care 2007;14:83–84.

Chapter 2
Medical Histories and Personal Protection

Aims

The first aim of this chapter is to examine the value of the patient's medical history in preventing the transmission of infection during dental procedures. The second aim is to look at personal protection of dental personnel.

Outcome

After reading this chapter, you should have an understanding of the use of the medical history and how personal protection is important in prevention of the transmission of infection.

Medical Histories

Taking an accurate medical history is essential before any dental procedure, but often is not helpful for determining whether a patient is an infection risk. This is because many of the potentially infectious diseases are "silent" – the patient may not know they have contracted them. Thus, unless the patient reports that they have been diagnosed as carrying a specific infectious disease, the medical history may not be helpful in determining their infectious status. Many potentially infectious diseases are associated with prejudice and stigma, notably HIV, and infected patients may as a consequence be economical with the truth in giving their medical history. In addition, in many countries, patients are not obliged by law to disclose information about certain infectious diseases they know they carry.

One frequently asked question in taking medical histories is to ascertain a history of jaundice. Although this question can be helpful in determining whether a person has liver disease, which can affect, for example, bleeding time, it is rarely helpful in eliciting liver infections, such as hepatitis B or C. A history of jaundice can also be unhelpful, because it could have been caused by hepatitis A or E, conditions which are usually self-limiting and do not pose an infection risk in dentistry. Jaundice is usually a late stage in the progression of hepatitis B and C infections. It is therefore unlikely that carriage of hepatitis

7

B or C would be elicited from a medical history, unless the patient has been diagnosed as having contracted them and reports them truthfully.

It is because the medical history may be non-contributory in determining whether the patient is an infection risk that standard precautions are used for all patients. Even if a patient does not report a significant diagnosed infection when the medical history is taken, if standard precautions are used, these should give protection against infection for all normal dental procedures.

Confidentiality

Any information given to a dental professional during a medical history must be completely confidential. All staff must be aware of this absolute need for confidentiality. Worldwide there have been a number of cases of breaches of confidentiality that have resulted in legal redress.

Infection Control Policy and Staff Training

Every dental practice should have a written and regularly updated infection control policy, which has been read and is adhered to by all members of staff (see Chapter 6 and appendices). It should be a condition of employment that all staff adhere to the policy. An example of an infection control policy is shown in Appendix 1. The policy should include a daily schedule of how to set up a surgery for various procedures (see Appendix 1). New members of staff should have full induction training in infection control (see Appendix 2) and should not learn just by observation during dental procedures. The compliance of all staff with infection control procedures should be regularly audited and discussed at practice meetings. In addition, all staff should periodically attend training sessions given by experts from outside the practice.

Pre-employment Health Checks for Dental Personnel

Countries vary in their legal requirements for pre-employment health checks for dental personnel. In some countries any personnel who have contracted HIV, hepatitis B, C or tuberculosis are prevented by law from doing, or assisting in dental operations. The evidence for preventing an untreated tuberculosis carrier from being involved in dental procedures is compelling, but after four weeks of a course of antituberculosis therapy they should not be any danger of transmission of infection. The case for barring a person who is infected with HIV is less conclusive, as highly active retroviral therapy should negate the very minimal risk of transmission. Many countries do not legally prevent HIV carriers from doing dental procedures, provided standard precautions are taken, appropriate medication used and regular health checks are done on the infected individual. Similarly hepatitis C has never been proven to be transmitted by dental personnel and it seems illogical to ban carriers from participating in routine dental procedures.

The main route for transmission of hepatitis B to dental personnel is from patient's blood on instruments after sharps injuries. It is probably related to the number of virions present in the blood. This can be assessed by estimating the number of hepatitis B DNA copies present in a unit of blood. Some countries recommend that dental personnel, if they are doing invasive dental procedures, should not have greater than 103 virions per ml present in blood but this condition is not universally employed.

The value of pre-employment health checks for HIV and hepatitis C is therefore questionable, but there is some merit in ensuring that carriers of hepatitis B and tuberculosis do not engage in invasive dental procedures.

Immunisation against Infectious Disease

Successful immunisation against infectious disease is an essential part of personal protection in dentistry. The immunisations that are commonly recommended are shown in Table 2-1 and cover a range of bacterial and viral disease. Many of the immunisations listed in the table are routine vaccinations against infectious disease given in most developed countries to infants or adolescents, and are not especially applicable to dentistry. Some of these vaccinations are not given routinely in some countries; a good example of this is tuberculosis. The use of an avirulent tuberculosis strain in the bacille Calmette-Guérin (BCG) vaccine has not been accepted by all countries, as its efficacy of protection and longevity has been questioned.

Barrier Protection

The hands, eyes and faces of dental personnel are the most vulnerable areas for the transmission of infection and should be safeguarded by barrier protection. Other areas such as dental clothing are more controversial.

Hands

The care of the hands is absolutely essential to all dental personnel. Emphasis should be placed on supple, intact skin with no cuts or abrasions and well-

Table 2-1 **Vaccinations recommended for dental staff**

Disease	Route	Length of protection
Diphtheria	Intramuscular	Probably lifelong if given in infancy, but some authorities recommend re-vaccination in adolescence
Hepatitis B	Intramuscular	Probably lifelong but some countries recommend re-vaccination every 5 years
Pertussis	Intramuscular	Probably lifelong
Poliomyelitis	Oral	Probably lifelong
Tetanus	Intramuscular	Probably lifelong
Tuberculosis	Subcutaneous	Protection can last for 15 years in some people, but is incomplete

cared-for nails and nail beds. This means that dental personnel have to care for their hands, not just while they are working, but at other times too. During hobbies which involve possible damage to the hands, such as gardening and car maintenance, the hands have to be protected.

A schema for the protection of the hands is shown in Fig 2-1. At the start of the day, the hands should be carefully examined and any cuts and abrasions covered with an adhesive waterproof dressing. It is essential that rings and watches are removed if detritus is not to accumulate under these items. Those who do not want to remove rings must completely cover them with waterproof adhesive coverings, but this is not ideal.

The hands can now be systematically washed and the easiest way to achieve this is to use a technique such as that described by Ayliffe and illustrated in Fig 2-2. The hands are first wetted all over, soap is applied and then the hands are washed using a systematic technique and then thoroughly rinsed. Careful rinsing is essential as soap draws water and oils out of the skin and if left in situ it can make the skin less pliable.

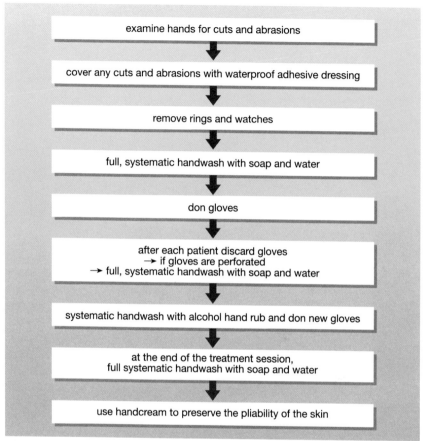

Fig 2-1 Schema for routine handwashing and protection.

The choice of soap is important and a personal choice. Bar soap should never be used as it can get heavily contaminated and can grow bacteria! Combinations of soap and disinfectant are effective, but often can damage the hands. Some soap and detergent combinations, such as those containing chlorhexidine, may contain chelating agents which may cause skin irritation, let alone stop the disinfectant from coming out of solution. The emphasis in initial handwashing for dental procedures is that the hands should be thoroughly cleaned; a disinfectant may be useful but is not essential.

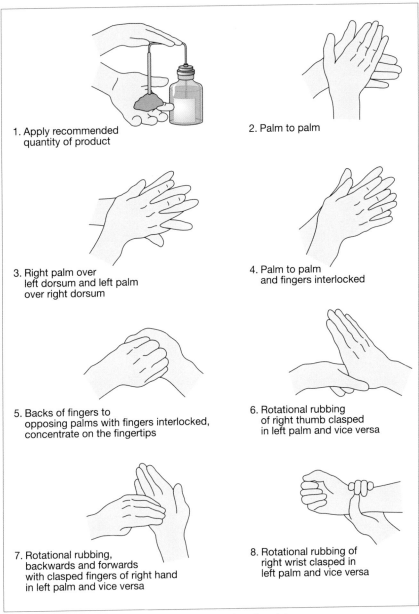

1. Apply recommended quantity of product

2. Palm to palm

3. Right palm over left dorsum and left palm over right dorsum

4. Palm to palm and fingers interlocked

5. Backs of fingers to opposing palms with fingers interlocked, concentrate on the fingertips

6. Rotational rubbing of right thumb clasped in left palm and vice versa

7. Rotational rubbing, backwards and forwards with clasped fingers of right hand in left palm and vice versa

8. Rotational rubbing of right wrist clasped in left palm and vice versa

Fig 2-2 The Ayliffe technique for systematic handwashing.

Everyone's skin is a little different and experimentation is necessary to find the optimum agent for personal hand cleaning. Once clean, the hands are thoroughly rinsed and carefully dried on disposable paper towels, avoiding abrasion. Thorough drying is important to avoid wet skin being trapped in gloves. This initial handwash is important and should not need to be repeated unless the operating gloves are damaged.

After each patient, the gloves are removed and the hands can be disinfected using an alcohol and disinfectant combination. Again the alcohol and disinfectant is applied using a systematic technique such as that shown in Fig 2-2.

At the end of the day the hands are systematically rewashed in soap and carefully dried. It is essential at this time to apply some emollient hand cream to prevent the hands from drying and to keep the skin pliant.

Hand Problems
Most of the problems dental personnel have with their hands manifest as simple inflamed areas. The commonest causes are:

- poor handwashing technique
- not covering retained rings properly
- soaps or disinfectants that react with the hands
- gloves with inherent chemicals that irritate the hands.

The most common type of inflammatory hand reaction is called irritant contact dermatitis (Fig 2-3). This can usually be cured by improvement of handwashing technique, change of washing agent, removal of rings or

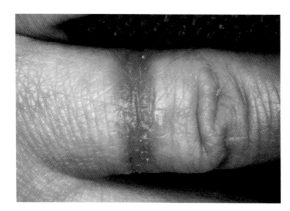

Fig 2-3 Irritant contact dermatitis, in this case caused by the non-removal of a ring.

13

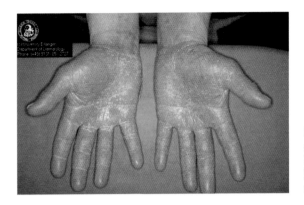

Fig 2-4 Allergic contact dermatitis. Courtesy of University of Erlangen Department of Dermatology.

changing the type of glove worn (see section on gloves below). Operators can react to alcohol and disinfectants, but this is rare. If irritant contact dermatitis is serious, then the help of a physician should be sought. Usually irritant contact dermatitis can be cured by a change of gloves, or washing agents, but sometimes the help of topical steroid preparations is necessary.

Irritant contact dermatitis is always limited to the hand area covered by the gloves. A more serious, and fortunately rare, skin reaction is allergic contact dermatitis, which is characterised by inflammation spreading well beyond the area covered by the gloves (see Fig 2-4). This is a hypersensitivity reaction, which is due to allergen(s) penetrating the skin and initiating a type 4 reaction. It can be very debilitating if it is chronic and will lead to breakdown of the skin, thus increasing the risk of acquired infection.

Rarely, a type 1 reaction can occur, leading to life-threatening anaphylactic reactions. All cases of allergic contact dermatitis need careful investigation and sadly, if the specific allergen cannot be identified, can lead to the cessation of dental operating. Allergic contact dermatitis is more common in those individuals with atopy.

Gloves

Dentists wear gloves longer than any other healthcare professionals, often for up to 8 hours every working day. It is therefore not surprising that problems such as irritant contact dermatitis and allergic dermatitis have been seen more often in dentists since the advent of glove use as barrier protection. There has been considerable debate about whether gloves can be reused after washing on multiple patients, but the consensus is that they are single-use items and should be discarded after every patient. Most gloves, even when unused, contain small microscopic holes, but these have not been shown to affect their barrier functions, or lead to infection.

Various materials are used to make gloves, including vinyl, nitrile, polychloroprene and elastyren. By far the most common are rubber or, more correctly, latex gloves.

Latex gloves were initially most favoured in dentistry because:

• they stretched and fitted well
• they could be made thinner for good tactile sensitivity
• they were relatively tough
• they were relatively cheap to make.

In Europe there are now strong moves to ban the use of latex gloves as they contain very powerful low-molecular-weight allergens. Exposure to these allergens has increased the incidence of latex allergy in the population and, in exceptional cases, has led to anaphylactic reactions in healthcare workers. Even if the gloves are carefully washed during manufacture, sufficient low-molecular-weight allergens remain to cause problems.

Most gloves also contain donning agents, which help the healthcare worker to put them on. One such agent is hydrogenated starch, as it is cheap. Its use cannot be too highly deprecated as it:

• spreads allergen into the atmosphere when the gloves are donned, which can be aspirated into the lungs and cause direct and indirect (allergenic) damage
• can cause adhesions in wounds
• can prevent the complete adhesion of fixed dental prostheses, crowns and veneers.

In many countries, gloves that contain deleterious donning agents have been banned from all medical and dental practice. However, hypoallergenic gloves are now available, which contain low quantities of protein. These suit many people and do not cause dermatitis. It is important to find a glove that suits you and your skin. This may mean experimenting with different types.

Eye Protection
Eye protection is essential during all operative procedures to prevent direct

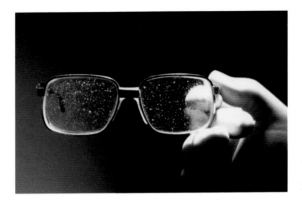

Fig 2-5 "Splatter" from the mouth can contain infectious agents.

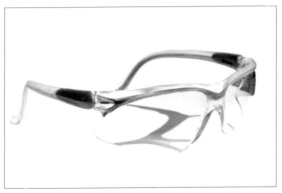

Fig 2-6 Eye protection.

traumatic injury. Traumatic eye injury can happen when, for example, old amalgam fillings are being removed and particles are "shot" out of the mouth at high speed.

Eye protection also shields against "splatter" from the mouth which may contain infectious agents (Fig 2-5). There is a variety of effective eye protection available. This ranges from visors to prescription spectacles (Fig 2-6). Eye protection is essential for the patient too!

Masks

These are not usually a microbiological protection, but are worn to prevent "splatter" and droplet infection from contaminating the face. Even good quality "theatre-type" masks rapidly become porous to micro-organisms when they are wet. Masks are a single-use item as they become contaminated during operative procedures and should be discarded after each patient.

Surgery Clothing

A whole variety of surgery clothing is available for dental procedures. Simple, routine dental procedures do not require elaborate sterile surgery clothing. There is little evidence to support the regular changing of surgery clothing between patients for routine dentistry. It is however essential that surgery clothing is not worn outside the surgery as it will be contaminated with saliva and blood.

Some authorities advocate long sleeves to prevent contamination of the arms. Others argue that an arm is easy to wash after a patient treatment, so that long sleeves are not essential. Many countries now favour short sleeves, as it facilitates good handwashing practices. What is perhaps more important is that surgery wear is clean and changed frequently as dentistry involves close contact.

The material used in surgery clothing is important. It should be capable of withstanding washing at 60°C as this temperature will reduce the microbial counts below a minimum infective dose on the garment.

Sharps Injuries

By far the biggest risk of infection during dental procedures are sharps injuries, where instruments contaminated with saliva penetrate the hands or other body parts. If the skin is fully penetrated then there is a real risk of blood-to-blood contact. Sharps injuries can occur at any time, but there are two occasions that are potentially most risky. The first is when needles are being resheathed following administration of local anaesthetic. The second is during the processing of used instruments.

Dentistry is the only part of the medical profession in which needles tend to be resheathed; most needles are discarded after single-use. Resheathing can be done safely by using one hand to hold the syringe and picking up the sheath from a hard surface by inserting the needle into the sheath. There are now a number of devices with inbuilt sheaths which allow safe resheathing.

Processing used instruments is also potentially a risk area for sharps injuries. Used instruments must not be manually washed (see Chapter 4) as this can lead to sharps injuries. When placing used instruments in washer disinfectors or ultrasonic machines, heavy duty gloves must be worn. A schema for the management of sharps injuries is shown in Appendix 1. All sharps injuries must be taken seriously and their reason analysed and suitable preventative measures taken.

Conclusions

- Medical histories do not always elicit whether a patient is a carrier of an infectious disease and standard precautions should always be adopted.
- Pre-employment health checks are important, especially to eliminate the risk of tuberculosis.
- Immunisation against a variety of infectious agents is important.
- Gloves provide good barrier protection.
- Eye protection during all operative procedures is essential.
- Masks are not a microbiological protection but should be worn to protect against splatter.
- Visors provide an excellent protective replacement for masks and glasses, when appropriate.
- Sharps injuries must be properly treated and prevented from recurring.

Further Reading

Field EA, Longman LP. Guidance for the Management of Natural Rubber Latex Allergy in Dental Patients and Dental Healthcare Workers. Good Practice Guidelines. London: FGDP(UK) RCSEng.

Smith AJ, Cameron SO, Bagg J, Kennedy D. Management of needlestick injuries in general dental practice. Br Dent J 2001;190;645–650.

ADA Council on Scientific Affairs. The dental team and latex hypersensitivity. J Am Dent Assoc 1999;130:257–264.

Chapter 3
Surgery Design and Surgery Equipment

Aim

The aim of this chapter is to delineate the principles for surgery design, which incorporate the principles of infection control. The selection of equipment is also discussed.

Outcome

After reading this chapter, surgery design and how it affects infection control, and the purchase of sterilisable instruments, should be understood.

First Principles

Very few dentists have the luxury of starting with a blank piece of paper and designing and building a dental practice. Most start with a building and convert it into a practice, which often means compromise. All too often infection control is an afterthought in the design and development of a dental practice.

The first major decision that has to be made is whether central decontamination facilities are to be used. The advantages of central facilities are the following:

- Instrument decontamination and processing is not done in the surgery.
- Steam and other emissions are confined to one area, with appropriate provision being made for ventilation.
- The noise from operating autoclaves, thermal disinfectors, ultrasonic baths and related equipment can be confined to one room.
- Machines for decontamination with high throughput can be used in centralised units.
- Only one decontamination facility has to be commissioned, tested routinely and validated.
- Testing, repair and maintenance of decontamination equipment does not interfere with clinical activities.
- It is possible to have suitably trained staff dedicated to delivering decontamination of appropriate quality.

There are, however, disadvantages to central decontamination facilities.

- The number of instruments required is high, as allowances have to be made for processing time.
- The capital cost of machines can be high.
- The cost of ventilation in the decontamination area can be high.
- Some surgery staff do not enjoy working full-time in instrument processing.
- Systems have to be designed for the safe transport of instruments to and from the surgery to the central facility.
- Central facilities can occupy a lot of space.

Central facilities are most efficient when a number of surgeries are being serviced from it. The best arrangement for central facilities is a "hub and spoke" design, with surgeries being provided with instruments from a directly contiguous central facility (Fig 3-1). This is seldom possible, so the safe transport of dirty instruments, in particular, has to be arranged in leak-proof containers or trolleys.

The position of the cleaning and sterilising equipment within the decontamination facility is also important (Fig 3-2). There should be a progress from dirty to clean areas with a sink in the dirty area to be used for decontamination. This sink must never be used for other purposes such as handwashing, let alone beverage preparation. Just before the sink there should be an illuminated magnifying glass to inspect the instruments. If instruments are still dirty after initial cleaning, then adherent material should be removed with a long-handled brush, with the operator wearing thick gloves, apron and eye protection. Beyond the autoclave should be a clean storage area.

If the decontamination process is undertaken in the surgery, then the designated area must be separate from the treatment area.

A schematic diagram of a suggested arrangement for a decontamination area in a surgery is shown in Fig 3-3. The process of cleaning and sterilisation is fully described in Chapter 4. Ventilation in areas used for decontamination has to vent externally and be powerful enough to remove steam and aerosols.

Cabinetry

Cabinets and work surfaces used in the dental surgery should be made so that they can be cleaned and will resist the use of surface disinfectants. Work

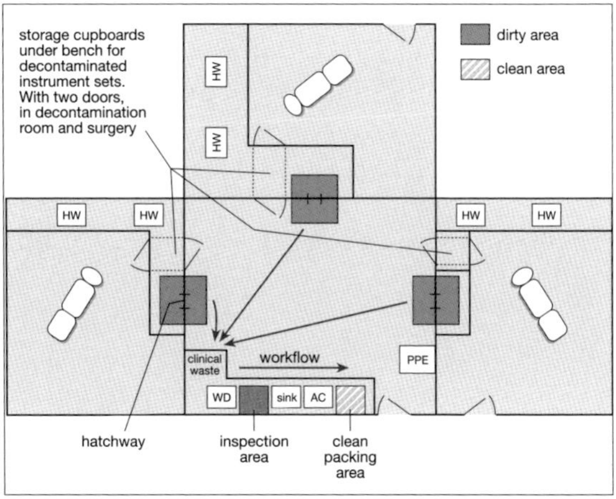

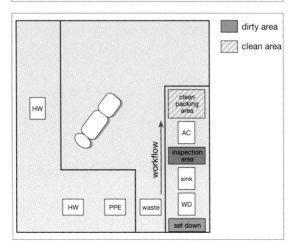

Fig 3-1 Possible design for "hub and spoke" layout for surgeries and central decontamination facility. HW = handwash sink; PPE = personal protection equipment; WD = washer disinfector or ultrasonic bath; AC = autoclave.

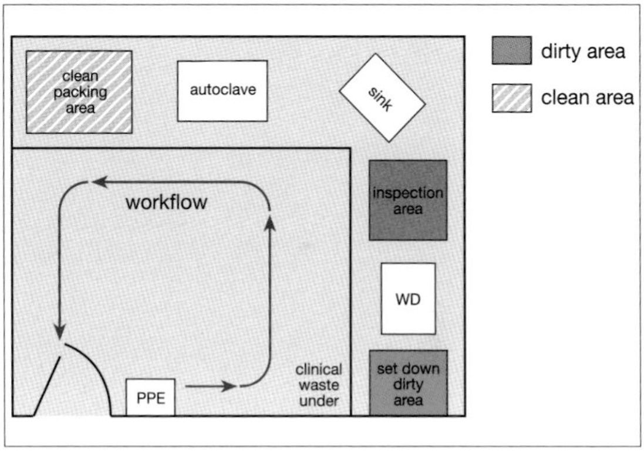

Fig 3-2 Possible layout of central decontamination facility with flow of work from dirty to clean areas. AC = autoclave; WD = washer disinfector or ultrasonic bath.

Fig 3-3 Schematic diagram showing possible layout of decontamination equipment within surgery. The decontamination area should be separated from areas of clinical activity. HW = handwash sink; PPE = personal protection equipment; WD = washer disinfector or ultrasonic bath; AC = autoclave.

21

surfaces should be free of clutter and not used to store instruments or materials. Keeping work surfaces clear makes the task of decontamination between patients a simple and quick process. Many modern surgery designs limit work surfaces to a minimum to reduce the area requiring decontamination, thus facilitating a rapid patient turnover.

Cabinets are used for single-use items, materials and aseptically stored instruments (trays, bags and pouches). Instruments should be stored in trays and kept inside cabinets until required. This minimises the risk of contamination prior to use.

It is not recommended to store clean instruments in bulk in drawers as they are at risk of contamination through contact with hands during clinical procedures. If cabinets and work surfaces are fixed, they should have sealed coving to eliminate gaps between the wall and floor and thereby prevent the accumulation of detritus.

Procurement of Instruments

The purchase of dental instruments must be done with infection control in mind. Two essential written pieces of information must be obtained from the manufacturer for any instruments.

• Is the piece of equipment single-use or capable of decontamination?
• What is the optimum method of decontamination?

There is an international standard, BS EN ISO 17664:2004, which sets out the requirements for manufacturers of medical devices to provide validated instructions on decontamination procedures for their equipment. These instructions should include preparation for cleaning, cleaning methods, sterilisation and storage requirements. It is a sad fact that only a small minority of reusable instruments are supplied with instructions on decontamination. Where instructions are provided, many do not comply with BS EN ISO 17664:2004. This makes it very difficult to comply with professional advice that manufacturers' directions should be followed.

Until regulatory authorities enforce compliance with these standards, this situation is unlikely to improve. Nonetheless, it is important when purchasing new equipment to ensure that it can be decontaminated satisfactorily, preferably using existing protocols.

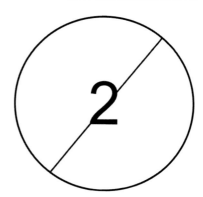

Fig 3-4 International symbol for single-use instruments.

Many surgery instruments are for single-use and have a symbol on them to this effect (Fig 3-4). These items must not be reused. The main reason why they are designated for single-use is that the manufacturer has deemed them not capable of reliable decontamination.

A large number of dental instruments are marked as for single-use, including matrices, endodontic instruments and saliva ejectors. Consideration should be given to making other items, such as burs, single-use, given the difficulty and cost of reliable decontamination. Instruments should not be purchased if there are uncertainties as to the appropriate arrangements for decontamination, or, in the case of single-use instruments, disposal.

Air conditioning

The role of airborne contamination in the transmission of infection in the dental setting is not well defined. Slit-samples of the air in dental surgeries have shown bacterial counts higher than normal background levels, in particular, when aerosols are being generated by equipment such as ultrasonic scalers and air turbine handpieces. Contaminated aerosols may be present in an area approximately two metres around the patient's head. Bacterial counts in this area may return to background levels within 10 minutes of completing procedures generating aerosols.

The movement of air in surgeries when doors are opened, or high-vacuum suction is used, helps disperse aerosols and reduces bacterial counts. Unless air conditioning incorporates high-efficiency particulate air (HEPA) filtration or electrostatic particle capture, it is unlikely to have much effect on microbial load. A major source of microbial air pollution is coolants for air turbines and powered scaling equipment. Effective high-volume suction during the use of such equipment can reduce pollution by over 90%.

Dental Units

There are a plethora of dental units available, all with differing designs. Before purchase, it is important to look at a dental unit with infection control in mind.

- Is the design likely to result in the accumulation of detritus in and around the unit?
- Is the surface of the unit capable of withstanding disinfection?
- Can the material for the patient's seat withstand cleaning and disinfection?
- Can the unit water supplies be disinfected (see Chapter 5)?

These are simple questions to which the manufacturer should be able to give written, evidence-based answers. Often examination of the unit will be reassuring or give cause for concern. More specialised elements of the equipment, for example, integral radiography machines or intraoral cameras, must be capable of being disinfected and cleaned.

Again, you must be satisfied by the manufacturer's information and your assessment of the acceptability of these items in terms of their ability to be cleaned and decontaminated.

Aspirators

Aspirators remove debris, blood, saliva and contaminated coolant water from the operative field. They must contain separators to remove particles, in particular, amalgam debris. The manufacturer must provide directions on the safe removal and disposal of separated material. Aspirators must vent externally, not directly into the surgery, to prevent contamination of the air.

Aspirators become very heavily contaminated as they collect infected material. They must be cleaned regularly to limit build-up of biofilm (see Chapter 5). Ideally, aspirators should be cleaned with a disinfectant and sur-factant combination (see Chapter 5). Again, before purchasing a dental unit, the manufacturer should give written directions on the cleaning and decontamination of the aspirator system.

Conclusions

- Surgery design must take account of infection control.
- Decontamination areas must have designated clean and dirty areas.
- Dental equipment must be provided with directions from the manu-facturers on cleaning and decontamination.
- Air conditioning and high-volume aspiration must vent externally.

Further Reading

British Standards Institution. Sterilization of medical devices. Information to be provided by the manufacturer for the processing of resterilizable medical devices. BS EN ISO 17664:2004. London: BSI, 2004.

Whitworth CL, Martin MV, Gallagher M, Worthington HV. A comparison of decontamination methods used for dental burs. Br Dent J 2004;197:635–640.

Bennett AM, Fulford MR, Walker JT, Bradshaw DJ, Martin MV, Marsh PD. Microbial aerosols in general dental practice. Br Dent J 2000;189:664–667.

Chapter 4
Instrument Decontamination

Aim

This chapter discusses the principles of instrument decontamination including cleaning, autoclaving and aseptic storage.

Outcome

After reading this chapter, you will understand how to operate a decontamination station and to check that it works safely.

Protocols and Training

Written protocols for decontamination of reusable instruments and for the safe disposal of single-use instruments must be produced. All staff involved in the treatment of patients and decontamination must be aware of these protocols and be trained in the use of the equipment involved. Records of training and regular updates should be kept.

Critical, Non-critical and Disposable Instruments

Before deciding how to decontaminate instruments, it is important to decide what instruments need to go through this process and which do not. Items such as the patient's protective glasses and bib chains do not normally get significantly contaminated with saliva or blood and are classified non-critical instruments. These non-critical instruments can be safely washed with detergent and dried before reuse.

The majority of instruments are significantly contaminated with saliva and blood and are called critical and need full decontamination. Some of the critical instruments are marked for single-use and must be disposed of safely. Other critical instruments are extremely difficult to clean effectively, for example, lumened instruments such as aspirator tips, which can be usefully replaced with typically relatively inexpensive, single-use items. Other critical instruments are complex in form, such as matrix bands and retainers, and decontamination may be time consuming and possibly present a risk of sharps injuries. Again, consideration should be given to replacing such items with single-use products.

As a general rule, difficult-to-clean and sharp instruments, which may pose a hazard to staff involved in handling contaminated instruments, should be disposable. Some national bodies may mandate some specific items of equipment as disposable; for example, in the United Kingdom, all endodontic files and reamers have been designated for single-use by the Department of Health.

Decontamination

The term decontamination is often thought, incorrectly, to just mean cleaning of instruments. Decontamination encompasses both cleaning and sterilisation and safe, aseptic storage. Places in dental surgeries where these functions are undertaken are often called decontamination stations. This chapter will discuss in detail how to operate, test and validate a decontamination station within a dental practice.

Choosing decontamination equipment
- Choosing equipment needs to be done with current and future needs in mind.
- The equipment needs to be fit for purpose and be designed and built to contemporary standards.
- Capacity should be at least adequate for current needs.
- In large practices, consideration should be given to buying several smaller capacity machines as opposed to a single, large machine. This will allow a degree of flexibility in the event of breakdown, routine maintenance and testing. It will also allow staggered cycle times to increase throughput.
- There should be good back-up arrangements in the event of malfunction and maintenance.
- There should be a training package included in the purchase of the equipment.
- Consideration should be given to leasing rather than purchasing equipment; this is often more cost effective and puts the responsibility for maintenance and testing on the supplier.

Instrument Cleaning
The first and most essential part of instrument decontamination is cleaning. If an instrument is not completely clean, then micro-organisms can be pro-

tected by adherent detritus from the sterilisation process and remain viable. The methods used for cleaning are manual, enzymatic agents, ultrasonics and washer disinfectors. The only safe and reproducible methods of cleaning are by means of washer disinfectors or possibly ultrasonic baths.

Manual cleaning of instruments

Hand cleaning of instruments is not effective or reliable. Even the most assiduous use of detergent, water and a brush does not completely, or reproducibly, clean dental hand instruments. Manual cleaning of instruments is also dangerous as sharp instruments are handled when they are maximally contaminated after use. Hand cleaning can be used for the removal of stubborn detritus after a mechanical process has been used, but appropriate precautions need to be taken.

Proteolytic agents

Proteolytic agents contain enzymes, which break down proteins and possibly split carbohydrates. They are useful for heavily contaminated instruments requiring a precleaning soak, in particular, if there is a lot of adherent organic material. Often containers filled with these enzymes are used as "holding tanks" prior to cleaning in a washer disinfector or an ultrasonic bath. This can prevent contamination from drying on the instruments, which makes removal all the more difficult. Proteolytic agents should not be used as a substitute for washer disinfectors or ultrasonic baths, but at most as an adjunct.

Ultrasonic baths

A common method for cleaning instruments is by means of an ultrasonic bath (Fig 4-1). This consists of a water bath to which is attached an ultrasound generating device (transducer). This sends sound waves through the liquid at frequencies of usually greater than 20,000 cycles per second. These sound

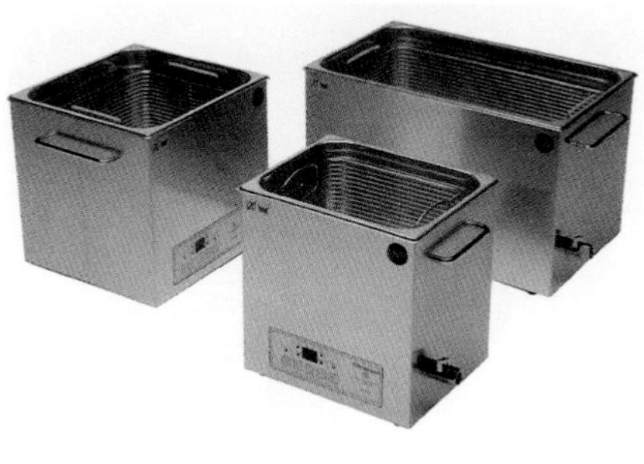

Fig 4-1 Common design of ultrasonic bath found in dental practice. Courtesy of Medisafe Ltd.

waves cause the liquid to flow back and forth in relation to the sound. An instrument immersed in the bath has liquid pushed towards it, then away from it under intense high pressure causing small "cavities" to form. The cavities are unstable and the liquid literally collapses against the instrument transferring energy to it and shaking it. It is this cavitation and transfer of energy that effectively lifts detritus from the surface of the instrument.

Ultrasonic baths work effectively if:

- they are properly commissioned before use
- they are tested periodically – at least every 3 months is usually recommended
- they are loaded appropriately
- they are used with a recommended detergent at the correct concentration and temperature
- they are used uninterrupted for the time recommended by the manufacturers
- they are fitted with a printout of the cleaning cycle
- the liquid is changed regularly and the internal parts of the tank scrubbed to remove adherent material – every three hours is usually recommended for general use, but more often if instruments cleaned in the bath are heavily soiled
- the users are provided with a written protocol on how to use the bath and have been trained in its use.

Before an ultrasonic bath is used the liquid in it needs to be degassed by starting the machine and running it without a load for the time recommended in the manufacturer's directions for use. The loading and operating time of an ultrasonic bath is critical.

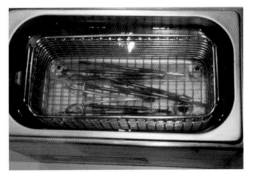

Fig 4-2 Correct loading of instruments in ultrasonic bath. There should be no overloading of the chamber, with space around each instrument; hinged instruments should be opened.

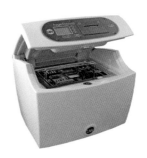

Fig 4-3 Ultrasonic bath with interlocking lid and printer displaying cycle parameters. Courtesy of Ultrawave Ltd.

Care must be taken not to overlap the instruments in the bath (Fig 4-2) and not to interrupt or add instruments during the cleaning cycle. Some ultrasonic baths are now fitted with a time lock to prevent cycle interruptions and a printer to record cycle parameters (Fig 4-3). Ultrasonic baths should be cleaned and dried when not in use.

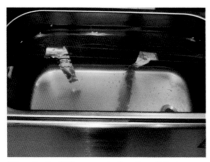

Fig 4-4a Ultrasonic bath with interlocking lid and printer displaying cycle parameters. Courtesy of Ultrawave Ltd.

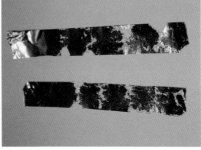

sFig 4-4b Foil ablation test strips demonstrating erosion pattern. Courtesy of Medisafe Ltd.

Testing an ultrasonic bath is usually done with strips of aluminium foil cut 20 mm wide and 10 mm long, suspended just above the bottom of the tank. The tank is first degassed and at least nine strips, weighted down with paper clips, are suspended just above the bottom of the tank with adhesive tape (Fig 4-4). The tank is then run for the manufacturer's recommended operating time and the strips removed and examined. The strips should show even corrosion. If there is no corrosion, then the sound transducers may not be working, or may have become detached from the bath.

Ultrasonic baths effectively remove blood and saliva from instruments, but are not effective in the removal of prions. Most ultrasonic baths are not suitable for cleaning dental handpieces. Some baths have irrigation devices in them, which aid in the cleaning of handpieces, but it is best to check with the manufacturer of the handpieces to be cleaned to ascertain whether ultrasonic cleaning is appropriate.

Washer disinfectors

Washer disinfectors are the preferred option for cleaning instruments before sterilisation (Figs 4-5 and 4-6). The reason is that, if properly commissioned, tested and validated, washer disinfectors clean instruments effectively, reproducibly and reduce the need for staff to handle contaminated instruments.

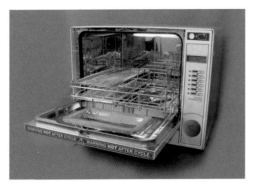

Fig 4-5 Benchtop washer disinfector. Courtesy of Medisafe Ltd.

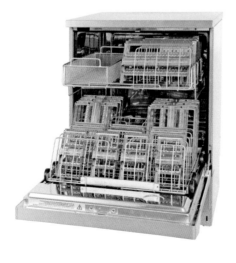

Fig 4-6 Large capacity, under-bench washer disinfector. Courtesy of Eschmann Ltd.

They do, however, require:

- between 25 and 60 minutes to cycle, which may mean that more instruments are required in the practice
- regular testing
- a source of clean water (see below)
- periodic revalidation.

They are also expensive to buy and to fit.
Washer disinfectors have five distinct processes.

- Initial flushing removes gross detritus from the instruments. Most now flush at <45°C which prevents most protein coagulation.
- A hot wash at about 60°C, using special detergents, removes any detritus. Washer disinfectors use detergents specified by the manufacturer. These detergents must be used according to the manufacturer's directions.
- Rinsing removes detergent and any remaining detritus, and is typically repeated several times.
- Thermal disinfection is incorporated into some machines. The temperature of the final rinse water is raised to a preset temperature and time, for example, 80°C for 10 minutes, or 90°C for 1 minute. The purpose is to kill most of any remaining micro-organisms.
- Drying removes residual moisture.

It is important to ensure that a washer disinfector is designed and built to appropriate standards and is fit for purpose. Accordingly, there are international standards for washer disinfectors (EN ISO 15883–1:2006). These standards include testing protocols. Therefore, when purchasing a washer disinfector, it is important to ensure that the manufacturer has a certificate of compliance with relevant international standards.

Washer disinfectors require commissioning according to manufacturer's directions, to ensure that they are functioning properly subsequent to installation. Regular testing is also required, again according to manufacturer's directions. In general, testing involves daily, weekly and quarterly tests.

Before starting each day:
- the spray arm should be checked to see that it moves freely
- spray nozzles should be cleared, as may be necessary, and the detergent reservoir filled
- the filters should be clean and clear.

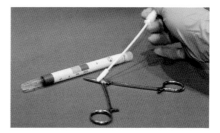

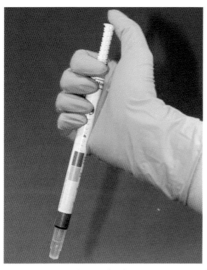

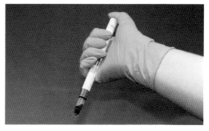

Fig 4-7a Simple residual protein-testing kit. Kit contains swab and reagent. Courtesy of Medisafe Ltd. **b** Swab is rubbed over surface of instrument to collect any residual protein. **c** Swab is submerged in reagent and colour is allowed to develop. The intensity of colour change is proportional to the amount of protein present.

Daily tests are done by operating the machine loaded and checking the display or printout to ensure that the manufacturer's parameters are reached for each part of the cycle. At the end of the cycle, the machine should give a visual indication that the cycle has been satisfactorily completed.

Every week, the washer disinfector should be tested to ensure that it is cleaning properly. This involves taking a representative instrument from a completed load and testing for traces of residual protein. Simple-to-use commercial kits are available for this purpose (Fig 4-7).

The cleaning efficacy of the machine should be periodically tested with a load that has been artificially soiled. The type of test varies from country to country, but they all use a "soil" that is applied to instruments. After the cleaning cycle, the instruments are checked for residual soil, usually using a protein test, the commonest being the ninhydrin method. This uses an indicator (ninhydrin), which changes colour if protein remains. A swab is rubbed over the contaminated instrument after cleaning, and any residual protein detected. Many other countries do not employ such a procedure. Records must be kept of all test procedures.

The water supplied to a washer disinfector must be chemically and microbiologically clean. Hard water needs to be softened to remove calcium salts, or the machine and detergent may not function optimally. Domestic water supplies often contain endotoxins, and, unless of potable standard, are unsuitable. The water demand of a washer disinfector can be high. One of the most practical ways of providing sufficient clean water is by connecting a reverse-osmosis machine to the water supply to the washer disinfector. These are readily available commercially.

Another method of providing sufficient clean water is by means of ion-exchange machines. These work well, but the quality of the water is not as good as with reverse osmosis. Both reverse-osmosis and ion-exchange machines must be properly commissioned and tested periodically.

Sterilisation
The preferred method of sterilisation after cleaning is by superheated steam. All other methods, including chemical immersion agents, are unreliable and must not be used.

Chemiclaves
These use a combination of microbiocidal chemicals heated to high temperatures. They are particularly useful for instruments that corrode when processed in steam.

There are, however, some disadvantages: it is imperative that they are serviced regularly and fitted with scavenger devices that effectively remove and prevent any trace of chemicals being released. In some countries the use of chemiclaves is subjected to very strict restrictions in respect of their siting and rigorous testing, making these devices almost impractical for routine use.

Autoclaves
Autoclaves employ water heated under pressure in a chamber, producing high-temperature steam. This superheated steam condenses on the surface of the instruments in the chamber, giving up its latent heat, rapidly raising the instrument's temperature to that of the steam. Any air pockets in the chamber or residual contamination on the surface of the instruments can effectively act as an insulator and prevent the rapid heating of the instrument, leading to failure of sterilisation.

It is important to ensure that an autoclave is designed and built to appropriate standards and is fit for purpose, according to relevant international standards

(BS EN 13060:2004), which include testing protocols. Autoclaves designed and built to comply with international standards will reliably self-test and "fail safe". It is very unlikely that such autoclaves will indicate the successful completion of a cycle, unless all the parameters are met. Therefore, when deciding on the purchase of an autoclave it is important to ensure that the manufacturer has a certificate of compliance with the international standards relevant to the model under consideration.

There are three types of benchtop autoclave suitable for use in a dental surgery.

Non-vacuum autoclaves (type N) displace air in the chamber by pumping in steam (Fig 4-8). These autoclaves are not suitable for wrapped or hollow instruments, but can work quite effectively on solid instruments.

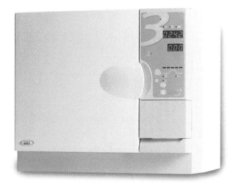

Fig 4-8 Typical benchtop type N autoclave. Courtesy of Prestige Ltd.

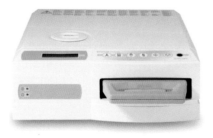

Fig 4-9 Cassette type S autoclave. Courtesy of SciCan Ltd.

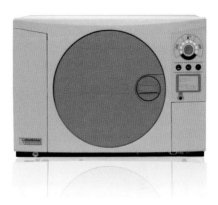

Fig 4-10 Modern benchtop type B autoclave. Courtesy of Eschmann Ltd.

Vacuum autoclaves (type S) have specific limitations on what instruments can be used in them (Fig 4-9). These displace the air in the chamber by pumping it out and then replacing it with steam. Vacuum autoclaves are effective when used within the manufacturer's range of parameters. This type of autoclave should be supplied with a list of instruments on which it has been tested and shown to be effective.

Vacuum autoclaves (type B) can be used with any hollow, wrapped or unwrapped dental instruments (Fig 4-10). These autoclaves have efficient vacuum pumps, which remove most of the air in the chamber and replace it with steam. These are by far the most versatile type of autoclave, but tend to have a longer cycle time than the other types of autoclaves.

All instruments should be dry and allowed to cool before they are removed from the autoclave. This helps prevent recontamination before reuse.

Ideally, all autoclaves should be fitted with a printout facility, which records the temperature reached and the time it was held. Some modern autoclaves have an internal memory and a computer interface that allows the cycle parameters to be downloaded and stored electronically. The temperature and time recommended for sterilisation in dental autoclaves is 134°C for 3 minutes at 2 bar pressure (2 atmospheres). Autoclaves are pressure vessels and have the potential to cause an explosion. The chamber, safety valve and door locks should therefore be regularly tested to ensure safe operation.

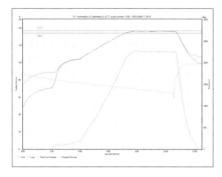

Fig 4-11a Thermocouple trace from N type autoclave. The green trace is from a thermocouple placed in the chamber above the load, the red trace is from a thermocouple placed within the load, and the blue trace is from a thermocouple placed in the chamber vent, i.e. the coolest part of the autoclave chamber. The purple trace is the pressure reading.

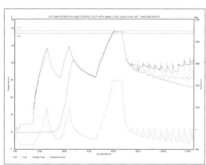

Fig 4-11b Thermocouple trace from B type autoclave. The green trace is from a thermocouple placed in the chamber above the load, the red trace is from a thermocouple placed inside a test load, consisting of folded towels to represent a porous load, and the blue trace is from the chamber drain, i.e. the coolest part of the chamber. The purple trace is the pressure reading. It should be noted that the heating-up part of the cycle alternates between vacuum production and admission of steam to replace the air removed from the chamber and load. Courtesy of Stericare Ltd.

Some autoclaves have "prion cycles" in their options for use. Prion cycles heat the contents to 134°C for 18 minutes, ostensibly to kill or inactivate prions. This temperature has no effect on prions and, as a consequence, prion cycles are not recommended.

Autoclaves are tested with indwelling thermocouples in various locations in the chamber (Fig 4-11). Most autoclaves include at least one fixed thermocouple in the chamber, usually in the coolest spot. This arrangement can be relied on to ensure that the required temperatures are reached. Autoclaves will show "cycle failure" on their display if the correct temperatures and holding time are not reached. If an autoclave cycle fails, it is usually a failure of steam to reach the required temperature during the holding time. The display will not indicate an overload of instruments in the chamber.

The water used to generate steam in autoclaves has to be free of protein and endotoxins and be soft. Most domestic water supplies are clean at the point of origin, but can be contaminated from storage in the building or being static in a system of pipes.

Domestic water supplies can become contaminated with low levels of Gram-negative non-enteric bacteria. These bacteria can become non-viable, lyse and release endotoxin from their cell walls. If the bacteria get into the water reservoirs of autoclaves, they can multiply and produce high counts and release endotoxins. For this reason, it is important that all autoclave reservoirs are cleaned thoroughly every day. Ideally autoclave water should be used only once, but older autoclaves recondense the used steam in the reservoir. For this reason it is important to drain and change reservoir water daily.

Some authorities recommend that "water for injection" should be used in autoclave water reservoirs. There is nothing wrong with this expensive practice, but the reservoirs must still be washed clean after every session. "Water for injection" is free of all impurities, including endotoxins. Distilled water or water passed through an ion-exchange system usually suffices for most autoclave systems. Such water can contain traces of endotoxin, but the concentrations are very small (fewer than 1 endotoxin units per ml) compared with the endogenous level in the mouth (240 units per ml).

Packing of instruments in the autoclave chamber is critical to whether the autoclave sterilises satisfactorily. Instruments should be placed in the autoclave in such a way that there is free circulation of steam around them. Overlapping instruments can cause failure of the sterilisation process. Hinged instruments such as forceps must have their beaks separated and the joint oiled. Wrapped and hollow instruments should not be sterilised in non-vacuum autoclaves as they may fail to sterilise. In addition, care should be taken to ensure that any instrument tray system is compatible with the selected autoclave and that periodic sterilisation checks are carried out.

Sterilisation checks
Autoclaves will register that the cycle has been satisfactorily completed, but this does not mean that instruments placed in the autoclave have been sterilised.

The autoclave will register that the cycle is complete if the indwelling thermocouple registers the correct temperature and time combination. The local conditions around an instrument in an autoclave determine if the instrument will be sterilised. This can vary with the position of the instrument in the autoclave, the packing and the way the steam circulates. It is impossible to check the sterility of every instrument subsequent to autoclaving. It is therefore important to be able to demonstrate that, if used correctly, conditions within the chamber will sterilise the load of instruments.

There are three main methods of checking sterility: thermocouples, or chemical or biological indicators.

Some large hospital autoclaves have the facility to place a thermocouple in any part of the chamber and to monitor the temperature externally and the time it is held. This is ideal, as it means the sterilisation of individual instruments in different positions, inside wrapping or on trays, can be monitored. Unfortunately, most bench-type autoclaves of the type used in dental surgeries do not have this facility.

Chemical indicators in the form of tubes, strips or incorporated on to the surface of bags or pouches are useful and convenient but have limitations. The chemicals in strips change colour when the sterilisation temperature has been reached but do not indicate that the temperature has been held for the correct time. They are therefore not a guarantee of sterilisation.

In some countries, biological indictors in the form of spore strips or tubes are used. They usually contain spores of *Geobacillus stearothermophilus*, formerly *Bacillus stearothermophilus*. The spores are usually contained in a small tube, which is put in an appropriate part(s) of the autoclave chamber. At the end of the sterilisation process, the tube is removed and growth medium released into it, usually by turning the screw cap, and the bottle is incubated at room temperature for up to 5 days. If the spores grow and sterility has not been achieved, then the indicator changes colour. *G. stearothermophilus* is a bacterium that lives in hot springs and is able to withstand much higher temperatures than most bacteria and, as such, finds application in assessing autoclave performance. It is of limited use, however, unless the instruments can be held in quarantine for the 5-day incubation period!

Aseptic Storage

Dental instruments, once sterilised, must be kept in aseptic conditions to prevent recontamination before reuse. For frequently used instruments, tray systems are by far the simplest and most efficient method of storage in primary dental care settings (Fig 4-12). Tray systems work well and can be colour coded for each dental operation. For instruments that are used less frequently, bags or pouches are very useful for storage. Many pouches are now made to allow the instrument to be seen and selected for use (Fig 4-13). Provided

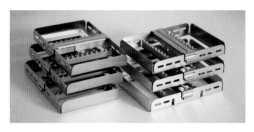

Fig 4-12 Tray systems suitable for use in washer disinfector and autoclave. Keeping instruments in sets in this type of tray minimises the handling risk to staff. Courtesy of Eschmann Ltd.

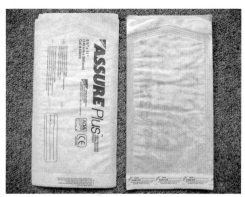

Fig 4-13 Clear pouch suitable for aseptic instrument storage.

instrument trays and pouches are dry and left undisturbed, then sterility can be preserved for considerable periods of time.

It is useful to write the date of sterilisation on the outside of the bag or pouch to enable a system of turnover to be used. Under no circumstances must instruments be stored in open drawers as they soon become contaminated by airborne and contact contamination. Similarly pouches, bags or trays stored when wet can allow the ingress of micro-organisms.

Handpieces

Dental high- and slow-speed handpieces can present difficulties in cleaning and sterilisation. Traditionally, handpieces were "cleaned" by squirting mineral oil under pressure through them. The handpiece is flushed with oil, with a napkin over the head until clean oil emerges from the lumens. This process only partially cleans the lumens and the complex architecture of the turbine blades.

Handpieces that have been oiled and subjected to autoclaving are not sterile. In addition when the handpiece has been cleaned with spray and autoclaved

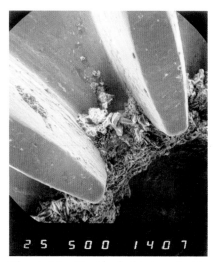 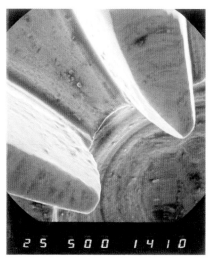

Fig 4-14a Residual detritus inside dental handpiece gearing after conventional compressed air cleaning. Courtesy of W & H Ltd.

Fig 4-14b Clean dental handpiece gearing after treatment with automatic handpiece cleaning machine. Courtesy of W & H Ltd.

many times, material becomes "baked" onto the turbine (Fig 4-14), its motion becomes eccentric, and this leads to wear, let alone trauma to teeth in preparation. Handpieces often need lubrication before and after sterilisation, causing contamination, as oil is not sterile.

Machines are available for cleaning handpieces more efficiently and effectively than simple spraying (Fig 4-15). These machines consist of either simple mechanical devices, which force detergent and oil sequentially through the inlet orifices of the handpieces, or more prolonged cleaning with a graded system of oils.

Handpiece cleaning machines are very effective. These machines are reported to prolong the satisfactory performance of handpieces and the life of the turbines.

Burs and Endodontic Files
Steel burs are exceptionally difficult to decontaminate and should be regarded as disposable. Diamond burs are more expensive, but are difficult to clean. The only reliable way to clean diamond burs is to remove the protein and

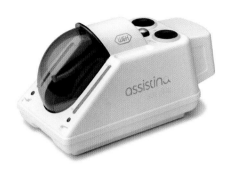

Fig 4-15 Automatic handpiece cleaning machine providing effective cleaning and lubrication. Courtesy of W & H Ltd.

other matter impacted on them with a proprietary proteolytic agent and then process them through a washer disinfector. Under such circumstances there is growing interest in single-use diamond burs.

Endodontic files are exceptionally difficult to clean because their design encourages protein and other material to adhere to them. They are also a frequent cause of sharps injuries to staff attempting to decontaminate them and as such pose a real hazard. In addition, as endodontic instruments may come into contact with neural tissue in the pulp and this could be contaminated with prions, these instruments should be single-use only. Many manufacturers mark their endodontic instruments as single-use.

Conclusions

- Decisions should be made as to which instruments are critical, non-critical or disposable.
- Many instruments are marked for single-use and these should never be reused.
- Instruments for reuse must be meticulously clean before sterilisation.
- Cleaning is best achieved with washer disinfectors.
- Ultrasonic baths, washer disinfectors and autoclaves must be properly commissioned and need careful, periodic testing to ensure that they are working correctly.
- Records should be kept of maintenance and testing of decontamination equipment.
- Staff involved in decontamination must be trained in the correct use of protocols and equipment. Records should be kept of such training.

Further Reading

British Standards Institution. Washer-Disinfection. Part 1: General Requirements, Terms and Definitions and Tests. European Standard EN ISO 15883–1:2006. London: BSI, 2006.

British Standards Institution. Small Steam Sterilizers. BS EN 13060:2004. London: BSI, 2005.

Chapter 5
Disinfection

Aim

This chapter explains what disinfection is and its uses in the surgery.

Outcome

After reading this chapter, you should have an understanding of the use of disinfectants on surfaces, drains, appliances and impressions and dental unit water supplies.

Disinfection

Disinfection is the removal or killing of some micro-organisms, but not usually spores. In hospital practice, the type of disinfection used is defined by three levels of risk.

- High risk is where there is a serious risk of transmission of infection. This is usually employed where patients have highly contagious infections, such as viral hæmorrhagic disease.
- Medium risk is where there is a real risk of transmission of infection. The disease is not as infectious but a risk exists.
- Low risk is where there is a risk of transmission of infection, but the chances are only slightly more than in normal life. Social washing, including hand-washing, probably negates this risk.

It is difficult to define the level of risk in dentistry, as there are few well-documented reports of transmissions of infection on which to base a judgement. Most routine dental procedures are thought by microbiologists to justify a medium risk, but this is a cautious approach.

The assessment of risk is important as it dictates what chemical disinfectant procedures are used and when. Chemical disinfectants can be used which, under certain circumstances, kill all cells with which they come into contact, including human cells. In dentistry, chemical disinfectants have to be chosen according to the risks encountered but that will not affect the operators. Disinfectants that can be used on skin or living tissues are called antiseptics.

45

Cleaning

The removal of dirt and fomites is an essential prerequisite to the process of disinfection. Many disinfectants are inactivated, or their efficacy negated, by the presence of dust or soil. Cleaning can be achieved by washing with a detergent, mopping or simply wiping with a damp cloth. It is important in a dental surgery to decide how areas are to be cleaned and when. Examples include the following.

- Floors are best cleaned with soap and water at the end of each surgery session. Cleaning surgery floors can release micro-organisms into the atmosphere and these need time to dissipate. Surgery floors should never be carpeted as they retain dust and dirt.
- Cabinetry surfaces and handles are best cleaned with soap and water at the end of each session. Working surfaces that will be used during dental procedures are disinfected after cleaning and before operating.
- Lights and dental chairs should be cleaned and disinfected after every patient.
- Sinks and taps should be cleaned with soap and water at the end of each session.
- Polythene covers are used to cover areas such as umbilical hoses for three-in-one syringes. They are effective if discarded after every patient but do not negate the necessity to clean.

Types of disinfectant

Some of the types of disinfectant available for dental purposes are shown in Table 5-1. The type of disinfectant used depends on risk. Most disinfectants have complicated modes of action, but in general have the following properties.

- They are selective in their action. Some, for example, are not good in acting against Gram-positive bacteria and viruses.
- They are inactivated by soil or organic matter.
- They are dependent on the pH of the environment.
- They are only stable for a limited period of time.
- They are time-dependent in their killing action.
- They all can have toxic effects.

It is of utmost importance that the deleterious effects of a disinfectant are assessed before use. The manufacturer's data sheets can help with this assessment. Written protocols should be given to all staff as to:

Table 5-1 **Types of disinfectant used in dentistry**

Disinfectant	Use
Alcohols	Hand disinfection and surfaces
Aldehydes	Surfaces but very toxic
Bisguanides (chlorhexidine)	Skin and hard surface disinfection
Hydrogen peroxide and other peroxygen compounds	Hard-surface disinfection, disinfection of DUWS
Iodine	Skin and hard-surface disinfection
Substituted aldehydes	Hard-surface disinfection
Triclosan	Hand disinfection
Quaternary ammonium compounds	Skin and hard-surface disinfection

DUWS = dental unit water supplies

- which disinfectant is to be used, where and when
- how each disinfectant is to be used
- what safety equipment must be employed when using the disinfectant
- what to do if any part of the body is exposed to the disinfectant.

Every member of staff must be given training in how to use disinfectants and be familiar with the relevant aspects of the surgery policy.

Surgery areas requiring disinfection

Disinfection is required in four distinct areas of the surgery:

- working surfaces
- impressions and appliances
- aspirators and suction devices
- dental unit water supplies (DUWS).

Working Surfaces

These are all the areas used during operating on a patient, including:

* the bracket table
* all handles and controls
* light handles and switches
* all equipment touched during operating.

These areas have to be cleaned and disinfected after use, given that they can become heavily contaminated with blood and saliva. The use of a spray-on disinfectant is recommended. This requires eye protection, and wearing heavy duty gloves and an apron to protect clothing. The procedure is as follows.

* Spray on disinfectant.
* Wipe vigorously with a clean cloth.
* Spray on disinfectant.
* Wipe off with a clean cloth.

This process cleans and dilutes the number of micro-organisms present to a level below a minimum infective dose. The risk from surfaces is low. Indeed there have been no reported transmissions of infection from surfaces in dentistry.

Disinfection of surfaces should be completed before the first patient arrives and after every patient, including the last patient of the session.

Impressions and Appliances

These must be disinfected before they leave the practice. Impressions are rinsed in cold, running water to remove any adherent blood or plaque and then immersed in a suitable disinfectant; spraying is inadequate. A number of immersion disinfectants suitable for all types of dental impressions are now available commercially that claim to cause minimal dimensional change.

It is important that impressions be rinsed carefully following the recommended period of immersion, as residual contamination affects the surface of casts and dies and may compromise the fit of the completed restoration or appliance. Appliances are treated similarly, with care being taken to ensure the disinfectant selected is not corrosive to any metal components of appliances.

The infectious risk from appliances is the subject of some debate. Some work has shown that the surfaces of appliances are minimally contaminated and the risk is small; there are, however, a number of contrary findings.

Aspirators and Suction Devices

These are heavily contaminated following use. Aspirator and suction tips should be single-use as reusable tips are nearly impossible to clean. Aspirator and suction systems collect large amounts of contaminated material and must be thoroughly cleaned and disinfected after every session. The internal surfaces of aspirator and suction tubing can become heavily contaminated with biofilm and, as discussed subsequently, need cleaning with a combination of a detergent/surfactant and a disinfectant. The detergent/surfactant disrupts the biofilm and allows the disinfectant to kill the residual micro-

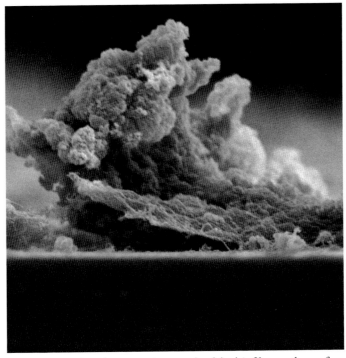

Fig 5-1 Scanning electron micrograph of the biofilm on the surface of dental tubing. Note the growth of bacteria and the small projections that spontaneously break off to release bacteria into the water. Courtesy of Optident Ltd.

Table 5-2 **Micro-organisms isolated from dental unit water**

Bacterial species	Fungal species	Protozoan species
Achromobacter xyloxidans	Alternaria	Acanthomoeba
Acineterbacter	Aspergillus	Cryptosporidium
Actinomyces	Candida	Giardia
Alcaligenes dentrificans	Penicillium	Microsporidium
Aeromonas	Phoma	Naegleria
Bacillus	Rhodotorula	
Bacteroides	Scopulariopsis	
Caulobacter		
Corynebacterium		
Enterococcus		
Flavobacterium		
Fusobacterium		
Klebsiella pneumophila		
Lactobacillus		
Legionella including L. pneumophila		
Micrococcus		
Moraxella		
Mycobacterium including M. avium		
Nocardia		
Pasturella		
Proteus vulgaris		
Pseudomonas including P. aeruginosa		
Burkholeria cepacia		
Streptococcus including Strep. mitis and salivarius		
Staphylococcus including Staph. aureus		
Xanthomonas		

organisms. A disinfectant that has strong cidal powers is recommended. Appropriate protective measures must be taken during these procedures. Aspiration and suction systems need cleaning after every operating session.

Dental Unit Water Supplies

DUWS can become heavily contaminated from micro-organisms in the water supply and from back-aspiration from turbines and slow-speed handpieces. The aspiration of micro-organisms from handpieces may occur, even if a back-aspiration prevention device is present in the line. The micro-organisms stick tenaciously to the walls of the tubing and form a biofilm (Fig 5-1). Micro-organisms in a biofilm can strongly resist the action of disinfectants, but are periodically released into the water supply to contaminate the coolant or irrigant water. The types of micro-organisms that are found in the DUWS are listed in Table 5-2. Potable drinking water must contain no enteropathogens – micro-organisms capable of infecting the gut – but these are commonly found in contaminated DUWS. Counts can be as high as several million in each millilitre.

DUWS must be initially purged to remove any biofilm present. This is done by running disinfectants into the system and allowing them to act for the recommended time. Disinfectants at either a lower concentration, or of a different type, are then introduced to prevent, on a continuous basis, more biofilm formation. Provision of clean DUWS is important as:
- infections can be spread by DUWS, in particular, in medically compromised patients
- legionellosis can be caused from contaminated DUWS – one practitioner has died as a result of such contamination
- endotoxin allergens from DUWS have been linked to late-onset asthma
- patients should have clean, potable water used in the provision of their dental care.

Conclusions

- Disinfectants should be chosen according to the risks involved.
- Surfaces, aspirators and suction systems should be disinfected after every session.
- DUWS need continuous disinfection to prevent the build-up of biofilm.
- Appliances and impressions must be disinfected before they leave the practice.

Further reading

Walker JT, Bradshaw DJ, Bennett AM, Fulford MR, Martin MV, Marsh PD. Microbial biofilm formation and contamination of dental-unit water systems in general dental practice. Appl Environ Microbiol 2000;66:3363–3367.

Smith AJ, Hood J, Bagg J, Burke FT. Water, water everywhere but not a drop to drink? Br Dent J 1999;186:12–14.

Chapter 6
Legal and Ethical Issues in Infection Control

Aim

To understand the ethical obligations of dental healthcare workers in the prevention of infection in the dental surgery.

Outcome

After reading this chapter, you should have an understanding of the need to behave in an ethical manner with respect to infection control issues. You will also understand the obligation to act within the laws that relate to the need to practise in a safe manner and environment.

Legal and Ethical Obligations

Although the law relating to infection control differs in detail around the world, it is usually contained within an overarching health and safety set of statutes. Dental practitioners each have an individual responsibility to practise in a safe manner, even though they may practise in a group or corporate environment.

Dental health professionals who fall short in their standards of infection control may be subject to action under either, or both, the criminal and civil legal systems. The state may prosecute persons who fail to provide a safe working environment and, if convicted, the penalties are often punitive, ranging from imprisonment to very large fines. Patients or staff who feel that they have been harmed as a result of inadequate infection control measures in their dental practice may bring a civil case for negligence.

In some countries it may not be necessary to prove that harm has been done, only that it may have occurred. It may be very difficult to refute such allegations without being able to robustly demonstrate compliance with the law and that professional guidelines have been strictly adhered to. It is not always necessary for a patient or member of staff to prove unequivocally that they contracted an illness through a dental procedure; it may be sufficient to show that on the balance of probabilities that an event occurred. This is made possible because the illnesses that can be transmitted often have long incubation periods, so proving cause and effect is often impossible.

Any conviction is liable to be brought to the attention of the national professional regulatory/licensing body and is therefore liable to jeopardise the future career of the health professional.

Ethics, on the other hand, are not contained within a framework of written laws, but are a set of guiding principles that should be followed to protect the integrity of the individual and the profession as a whole. Dental practitioners have a duty of care to protect the health and well-being of their patients and employees; proper infection control is fundamental to this duty. There is a public expectation that patients will be treated in a safe environment and their treatment will be delivered to as high a standard as possible, and that their general health will not be compromised by dental treatment. The general public have come to expect ever higher standards often fuelled by "scare stories" in the media. The hysteria that surrounded the emergence of AIDS in the 1980s led to fears that transmission could occur during dental treatment, even though there was no evidence of this, with a single exception in the USA (see Chapter 1). There was, however, as a result of this event a heightened awareness of the need to practise good standards of infection control in dentistry.

Standards have risen inexorably since that time, often with the dental profession feeling that there was not a sufficient evidence base behind the changes. Nevertheless, guidance on matters relating to infection control are reviewed and updated regularly by professional bodies and national health agencies.

Dental practitioners have an ethical duty to follow this guidance and to keep themselves updated through postgraduate education and training. This is now a formal requirement by Dental Councils and Boards; for example, the United Kingdom's General Dental Council makes it a mandatory requirement for its registrants to carry out a certain number of hours of decontamination training within a continuing professional development cycle.

There appears to be an increasing number of cases seen by regulatory bodies' disciplinary committees that are centred on allegations of poor infection control measures. This may continue to be a trend with a greater public perception of the importance of infection control.

Dental healthcare workers who suspect that they have an infectious disease have an ethical duty, for the protection of themselves, colleagues and patients, to seek and to follow medical advice. In some countries, this may mean a temporary or permanent end to their clinical practice and, as a consequence, does not encourage the necessary action.

Nevertheless, failure to act is indefensible.

To begin to defend any allegation of poor infection control, it is important to be able to demonstrate that robust policies and protocols are in place. These should be written and must be reviewed at regular intervals, at least annually, and must contain the essential elements of national and professional guidance. Equally important is the ability to demonstrate that all members of the dental team are appropriately trained in the principles of infection control and are able to implement all relevant policies and protocols.

In most countries, it is considered unethical to refuse to treat patients who have a known infectious disease, and may lead to accusations of discrimination. It is also unnecessary to treat such patients any differently to other patients; for example, at one time it was common practice to treat hepatitis B infected patients at the end of the day and to take special precautions. This is now considered to be untenable as standard precautions should take care of the risks posed by these patients, let alone others who do not know they are infected.

Discriminating against patients may make them reluctant to reveal their medical status. This can lead to complications in other respects for their dental care. It may be justified, however, to postpone elective treatment for some patients until their infective risk is reduced, for example, patients with acute herpetic lesions or tuberculosis.

At present, in view of the enormous uncertainties surrounding the inactivation of prions, it may be prudent to refer patients suspected of having Creutzfeldt-Jakob disease for treatment in a specialist unit that has ready access to an incinerator for the safe disposal of contaminated instruments.

Policies and Protocols

These should be written and available to all staff. It is good practice to issue personal copies to all employees and to get them to sign to acknowledge that they have received and read them.

It is often not necessary to have to invent new documents, as professional bodies often produce model documents that can be accessed and personalised for use in specific workplaces. Examples of the contents of practice policies and protocols can be found in the appendices.

It is good practice to appoint an appropriately trained member of staff as an "infection control supervisor". The roles of such a person may include:

- taking a lead role in all matters relating to practice infection control
- producing written policies and protocols and ensuring they are regularly reviewed and updated
- being responsible for all staff training in infection control, including induction training, update training and maintaining training records
- ensuring that all staff comply with infection control policies
- ensuring that staff vaccinations are updated and recorded
- ensuring an appropriate quality assurance scheme is in place
- ensuring that decontamination equipment is properly maintained, validated, tested and records kept
- ensuring that adequate supplies of personal protective equipment are available and that staff know how to use them
- liaising with the person responsible for equipment procurement to ensure that it can be decontaminated using practice protocols
- investigating all incidents involving potential infection risks, for example, sharps injuries
- ensuring that appropriate action is taken and recorded and that learning from such incidents is disseminated to all staff.

Training

Training in infection control within a practice is extremely important. It should be robust and effective. It is important that training needs are assessed for all members of the dental team and appropriate training is delivered, taking account of individual needs and requirements. All staff must understand their individual responsibilities for the safety of themselves, other members of staff and members of the public.

All members of staff should have an understanding of the causes of infections, how they are spread and the methods for controlling them. For some staff that may mean basic hygiene training; other staff, depending on their duties within the surgery, will need a more detailed understanding of infection control. Staff responsible for operating decontamination equipment should be fully trained in the use of the equipment. All new staff must have induction training before they are allowed to work in the surgery environment.

Training can be provided in a variety of ways – through one-to-one instruction by the infection control supervisor, by attending postgraduate lectures, by reading books, journals or guidance documents, by engaging the services of in-practice third-party trainers, or through computer-based training programmes. The suppliers of decontamination equipment should include staff training as a part of the commissioning process for all new equipment. It is important that the level of attainment of all staff receiving training is assessed and documented.

As previously stated, it is important that all staff training is recorded; for example, a record can be kept in each member of staff's personal file in the practice. Such records can be a very valuable piece of evidence should an allegation of malpractice, involving infection control, be made against the practice.

Conclusion

It is an absolute duty of all members of the dental team to ensure that they adopt policies and procedures that will minimise the risk of cross-infection occurring within the dental environment.

Further reading

There are no specific references on this subject. You are referred to the specific infection control guidelines of your dental association and of Fédération Dentaire Internationale (FDI). Many indemnity organisations provide detailed advice to their members on the ethical issues surrounding infection control.

Model Policies, Protocols and Checklists

Infection Control Policy

Good infection control is central to the safe running of this dental practice. Any failure to implement and comply with this policy can jeopardise the health of ourselves, our families and our patients. Any member of staff not complying with this policy will be subject to disciplinary action. All members of staff will receive infection control training appropriate to their duties. No member of staff may carry out procedures or operate equipment unless they have received appropriate training.

[Name] .... is the designated infection control supervisor (ICS) for this practice and is responsible for all infection control issues. Any accident involving potentially infected equipment or materials or decontamination equipment malfunction must be reported to the ICS. If any part of this policy is unclear, please discuss it with the ICS.

Personal Protection
- All members of staff must be appropriately vaccinated, including vaccination for hepatitis B. A record will be kept of vaccinations, including hepatitis B immunity status.
- Personal protective equipment (PPE) is provided for all staff, appropriate to their duties. This includes gloves, eyewear, masks/visors and protective clothing, which must be worn by all staff engaged in clinical procedures, including instrument decontamination. Protective clothing worn in clinical areas, including the decontamination areas, must not be worn outside the practice.
- Hand hygiene is extremely important. Hands must be washed using .... [soap product] and may be decontaminated using .... [alcohol gel]. Gloves must be worn for all clinical procedures, including decontamination. Gloves must be changed after each patient and and when damaged. If you have any reaction to either hand-hygiene products or gloves this must be reported to the ICS. Rings and watches must be not be worn during operating sessions to facilitate good hand hygiene.

- All inoculation injuries must be reported immediately to the ICS and recorded in the practice incident book. Immediate action should be to encourage the wound to bleed, washing under running water, followed by covering with a waterproof dressing. Further advice and actions can be found in the practice sharps injury protocol.
- Needles must be kept sheathed when not being used. Resheathing of needles must only be done using a resheathing device.

Decontamination of Equipment
- All reusable equipment must be decontaminated, as soon as possible, according to the practice decontamination protocol, and before use on a further patient.
- Decontaminated instruments must be stored in covered trays and/or pouches.
- All equipment marked or designated single-use must never be reused and must be disposed of in the appropriate clinical waste container.

Environmental Cleaning
- All work surfaces should be kept clear to facilitate cleaning.
- Clean instruments and materials must not be stored on work surfaces, where they may become contaminated.
- Areas that may be potentially contaminated during treatment should be clearly identified and kept to a minimum. After each patient treatment these areas will cleaned using ....
- All contaminated waste will be disposed of according to the practice clinical waste protocol.
- All clinical waste will be stored in .... until collected for disposal.
- All impressions and appliances must be rinsed under cold running water until visibly clean and disinfected by immersing in ....
- Any spillages involving blood or saliva will be reported to the ICS.

Author.................................. Date..

Review date .... [at least annually].

[Suggested protocols are generic and intended to include essential features. The details within these protocols will depend on local, national or international standards, regulations and guidelines. Where there are optional methods, these are included, but those that do not apply to a particular situation should be omitted from the adopted protocol.]

Decontamination protocol

All reusable instruments in this practice will be decontaminated using this protocol before further use.

- Contaminated instruments must be cleaned as soon as possible after use. If there is likely to be a delay, which could lead to debris drying on to the instruments, the instrumentation should be stored submerged in a freshly made solution of .... [enzymatic cleaner] until processing occurs. This should not exceed a period of 2 hours.

Washer Disinfectors
- At the beginning of each day, an automatic control test must be carried out, according to the manufacturer's directions.
- Contaminated instruments must be carefully loaded into the washer disinfector chamber paying particular attention to the correct loading pattern detailed in the manufacturer's directions for use.
- When the load is complete, the machine is switched on ensuring the correct cycle is selected.
- When the cycle is complete the display/printout must be checked to ensure that a successful cycle has been completed.
- If the machine indicates a failed cycle, the process must be repeated until a successful cycle is indicated.
- In the event of a malfunction of the machine, this must be immediately reported to the ICS.

Ultrasonic Baths
- At the beginning of each clinical session the bath should be filled to the correct level★ with .... [ultrasonic cleaning solution].
- The machine must be run for ..... minutes★ to degass the solution before use.
- Contaminated instruments should be carefully loaded into the bath, paying particular attention to the correct loading pattern detailed in the manufacturer's directions for use.
- The lid must be placed on the machine before switching on.
- The machine is then switched on, ensuring the correct setting is selected for ..... minutes★.

UNDER NO CIRCUMSTANCES MUST THE CYCLE BE INTERRUPTED.

- At the end of the cycle, the instruments must be carefully rinsed in .... [state type] water.
- If at any time the ultrasonic cleaning fluid appears to be visibly contaminated, it must be changed.

Instrument Inspection
- Wet instruments must be dried using a clean, disposable, lint-free cloth before inspection for cleanliness.
- Instruments must be inspected for visible cleanliness using illuminated magnification before continuing to sterilisation.
- Any instruments that are not visibly clean must be reprocessed through the cleaning cycle until clean. Traces of stubborn dental materials can be carefully removed manually using .... [for example, a metal-bur-type brush].
- Repeated failure of the equipment to clean adequately must be reported to the ICS.

Sterilisation
- Cleaned and dried instruments are carefully loaded into the autoclave chamber, ensuring there is sufficient space between instruments to allow for the free circulation of steam.
- Select the correct cycle .... [for example, 134°C for 3 minutes] and switch on the autoclave.
- When the cycle is complete, the indicator on the machine/printer should be examined to ensure that the cycle was successful. If there is an indication of a failed cycle, all instruments in the load must be recycled until a cycle is confirmed as satisfactory. Repeated fault/failure of autoclave cycles must be reported to the ICS.
- At the end of the successful cycle, allow instruments to cool and dry before removing them from the autoclave.

Storage
- Sterilised instruments must be stored immediately in .... [a covered environment] to prevent the possibility of recontamination before further use.
- Instruments that may have a prolonged period of storage before reuse should be stored in sealed pouches.
- Other instruments should be used as soon as possible after sterilisation.

★ *See manufacturer's recommendations.*

Model Protocol for Maintenance and Testing of Decontamination Equipment

All new decontamination equipment installed in this practice will be appropriately* commissioned before being released to the ICS for general use.

Testing, maintenance and repair records of all decontamination appliances in the practice are the responsibility of the ICS. Any malfunctions must be immediately reported to the ICS.

Washer Disinfectors
- Regular maintenance of the washer disinfector(s) is important and should be carried our every .... [interval*] months.
- Daily checks:
  - All water jets clear
  - Spray arms move freely
  - Door lock function
  - Detergent level (and salt).
- Daily testing – automatic control test (see manufacturer's recommendations)
- Weekly testing – residual protein test on processed instrument(s)*
- .... [Interval]-monthly soil challenge test.*

Ultrasonic Baths
- Ultrasonic cleaning fluid must be changed every session.
- Daily monitoring of the correct temperature and level of fluid.
- .... [Interval*]-monthly foil-ablation test.

Autoclave
- Fill water reservoir.
- Check waste water reservoir empty (if fitted).
- Daily automatic control test.
- Periodic validation testing*.

★ *Refer to local/national/international guidelines and manufacturer's recommendations.*

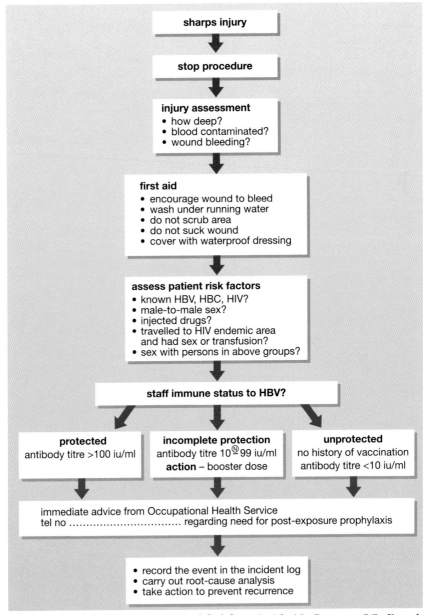

Fig A-1 Sharps injury protocol. Modified from Smith AJ, Cameron SO, Bagg J, Kennedy D. The management of needlestick injuries in general dental practice. Br Dent J 2001;190:645–650.

Suggested Components of Sharps Injury Protocol (see Fig A-1)

- Involvement of ICS as soon as possible
- Staff training
- First aid procedures
- Definition of "significant exposure"
- Assessment of risk status of patient
- Source of emergency occupational health advice at all times
- Access to post-exposure prophylaxis (PEP) drugs
- "Significant incident" reporting arrangements and root-cause analysis
- Record keeping.

Daily Infection Control Checklists

At the start of the day:

- Check washer disinfector/ultrasonic bath chemicals.
- Perform daily washer disinfector and autoclave checks.
- Run automatic control tests on washer director and autoclave.
- Fill autoclave water reservoir.
- Fill dental unit water reservoir.
- Peform systematic handwash.
- Thoroughly decontaminate all work surfaces.

Before each patient treatment:

- Ensure all equipment has been decontaminated.
- Use disposable coverings for surfaces likely to become contaminated.
- Set out equipment and materials for procedure.
- Decontaminate hands.
- Put on eye protection, masks, gloves etc.
- Provide eye protection and protective cover for patient.

During patient treatment:

- Change gloves if damaged.
- Use rubber dam where appropriate.
- Use high-volume aspiration when using turbine handpieces and ultrasonic scalers, starting the aspirator before reusing the handpiece or scaler.
- Handle sharps carefully; only resheath needles using a safety device.
- Clean dental materials from instruments during treatment.

After patient treatment:

- Dispose of sharps in sharps container.
- Segregate and dispose of clinical waste.
- Decontaminate all work surfaces that have been contaminated.
- Clean and disinfect impressions and appliances before dispatch to the laboratory.
- Place all instruments in washer disinfector/ultrasonic bath/holding solution.

- Remove and dispose of gloves.
- Decontaminate hands.
- Write up clinical notes.

At the end of the session:

- Decontaminate all work surfaces thoroughly.
- Disinfect aspirator unit and spittoon.
- Clean dental chair and unit.
- Empty ultrasonic bath (if applicable) and leave to dry.
- Empty autoclave waste water reservoir (if fitted).

At the end of the day:

- Drain autoclave water reservoir and waste water reservoir (if fitted).
- Disinfect dental unit water system and leave water reservoir to dry.
- Remove all clinical waste from surgery area and store in safe designated area, to await collection.

Appendix 2
Syllabus for Infection Control Training for Members of the Dental Team

Induction Training for all Staff

Induction training should include:

- basic principles of the spread of infection
- confidentiality
- understanding the practice infection control policy
- roles and responsibilities of the practice infection control supervisor
- hand hygiene and care
- importance and correct use of personal protective equipment
- personal protection, including vaccinations.

Additional Training for Clinical Staff

Additional training should include:

- decontamination of surgery environment, including work surfaces, dental unit water systems and suction systems
- decontamination of instruments
- safe storage of sterilised instruments and equipment
- disposal and storage of clinical waste
- sharps injury policy.

Training for Staff involved in Decontamination of Reusable Instruments

Training should include:

- importance of cleaning instruments before sterilisation
- operation of instrument-cleaning equipment, including correct loading
- operator testing of instrument-cleaning equipment
- recognition of instrument-cleaning equipment malfunction and action to be taken

- daily maintenance of instrument-cleaning equipment
- inspection of instruments following cleaning
- principles of sterilisation
- safe operation of autoclaves, including correct loading
- operator testing of autoclaves
- recognition of autoclave malfunction and action to be taken
- daily maintenance of autoclaves
- safe storage of sterilised instruments
- importance of daily checks and record.

Index

Quintessentials of Dental Practice Series

in 44 volumes

Editor-in-Chief: Professor Nairn H F Wilson

The Quintessentials of Dental Practice Series covers basic principles and key issues in all aspects of modern dental medicine. Each book can be read as a stand-alone volume or in conjunction with other books in the series.

Clinical Practice, Editor: Nairn Wilson

> Culturally Sensitive Oral Healthcare
> Dental Erosion
> Special Care Dentistry
> Evidence-based Dentistry
> Infection Control for the Dental Team

Oral Surgery and Oral Medicine, Editor: John G Meechan

> Practical Dental Local Anaesthesia
> Practical Oral Medicine
> Practical Conscious Sedation
> Minor Oral Surgery in Dental Practice

Imaging, Editor: Keith Horner

> Interpreting Dental Radiographs
> Panoramic Radiology
> 21st Century Dental Imaging

Periodontology, Editor: Iain L C Chapple

> Understanding Periodontal Diseases: Assessment and
>   Diagnostic Procedures in Practice
> Decision-Making for the Periodontal Team
> Successful Periodontal Therapy: A Non-Surgical Approach
> Periodontal Management of Children, Adolescents and
>   Young Adults
> Periodontal Medicine: A Window on the Body
> Contemporary Periodontal Surgery: An Illustrated Guide
>   to the Art Behind the Science

Endodontics, Editor: John M Whitworth

> Rational Root Canal Treatment in Practice
> Managing Endodontic Failure in Practice
> Adhesive Restoration of Endodontically Treated Teeth

Prosthodontics, Editor: P Finbarr Allen

> Teeth for Life for Older Adults
> Complete Dentures – from Planning to Problem Solving
> Removable Partial Dentures
> Fixed Prosthodontics in Dental Practice
> Applied Occlusion
> Orofacial Pain: A Guide for General Practitioners

Operative Dentistry, Editor: Paul A Brunton

> Decision-Making in Operative Dentistry
> Aesthetic Dentistry
> Communicating in Dental Practice
> Indirect Restorations
> Dental Bleaching
> Dental Materials in Operative Dentistry
> Successful Posterior Composites

Paediatric Dentistry/Orthodontics, Editor: Marie Therese Hosey

> Child Taming: How to Manage Children in Dental Practice
> Paediatric Cariology
> Treatment Planning for the Developing Dentition
> Managing Dental Trauma in Practice

General Dentistry and Practice Management, Editor: Raj Rattan

> The Business of Dentistry
> Risk Management in General Dental Practice
> Quality Matters: From Clinical Care to Customer Service

Dental Team, Editor: Mabel Slater

> Team Players in Dentistry

Implantology, Editor: Lloyd J Searson

> Implantology in General Dental Practice

Quintessence Publishing Co. Ltd., London

76